Take Away Insomnia And Restore Your Rest

A Comprehensive Guide To Managing Insomnia For Adults From Age 18 To 40

Nora B. Payne

This book is intended to provide general information only. The author and publisher have made every effort to ensure the accuracy of the information herein.

Table Of Contents

Purpose of this Guide

My friend, Martha, used to suffer from insomnia in the past, this always drove me crazy until we found a nice solution for her

This book seeks to give a complete overview of insomnia and equip young adults aged 18 to 40 with practical solutions for controlling this sleep problem. The book dives into the definition, causes, symptoms, prevalence, and impacted demographics of insomnia, trying to enable individuals to detect and solve their sleep troubles.

The book presents a range of evidence-based treatments and therapies for controlling insomnia, including lifestyle adjustments, cognitive-behavioral therapy, pharmaceutical interventions, and home remedies. It allows readers to take charge of their sleep health, gain a better awareness of their sleep patterns, and make educated decisions to encourage restful sleep and increase their quality of life.

The book also supports holistic well-being, acknowledging the interdependence of sleep with physical, mental, and emotional health. By addressing underlying issues leading to insomnia and encouraging healthy sleep habits, readers may nurture overall well-being and resilience in handling life's obstacles.

Introduction

Insomnia, frequently defined as the difficulty of getting asleep or staying asleep, is a widespread sleep problem that affects individuals across many age groups. In this thorough guide, we will dig into the concept of insomnia, investigate its underlying causes, address frequent symptoms experienced by individuals, and study its incidence and impacted demographics, with a special focus on young adults aged 18 to 40.

Definition of Insomnia

Insomnia is a sleep condition defined by persistent difficulties in beginning or sustaining sleep, despite enough chances for sleep. Individuals with insomnia generally experience unhappiness with the quality or amount of their sleep, leading to daily impairment and misery. It is vital to differentiate between acute insomnia, which lasts for a brief length and is generally prompted by stress or life events, and chronic insomnia, which persists for at least three nights per week for three months or more.

Explanation of the Disease

The underlying processes of insomnia are diverse and might differ across individuals. Factors leading to insomnia may include psychological stress, anxiety, depression, irregular sleep patterns, poor sleep hygiene, medical diseases such as chronic pain or respiratory illnesses, substance use, and certain medicines. Additionally, abnormalities in the body's circadian rhythm, which governs the sleep-wake cycle, can play a significant role in the development and maintenance of insomnia.

Common Symptoms

Individuals with insomnia may suffer a range of symptoms that influence their sleep quality and daytime performance. Common symptoms include difficulty falling asleep, waking up often during the night, difficulty remaining asleep, getting up too early in the morning, non-restorative sleep, daytime weariness, irritability, difficulty focusing, and poor performance at work or school.

These symptoms can lead to severe distress and impairment in numerous aspects of life, compromising overall well-being and quality of life.

Prevalence and Affected Demographics

Insomnia is a major sleep problem, affecting millions of persons worldwide. According to epidemiological research, roughly 30% of individuals have symptoms of sleeplessness, with various degrees of severity. While insomnia can occur across all age ranges, particular subgroups may be more vulnerable to developing insomnia. Young adults, particularly those between the ages of 18 and 40, are at higher risk due to lifestyle variables, academic or vocational stress, and changes in sleep patterns associated with transitions such as starting college or joining employment.

Furthermore, evidence shows that insomnia is more widespread in women than in men, with hormonal changes, pregnancy, and menopausal symptoms leading to sleep difficulties in females. Additionally, those with pre-existing mental health issues such as anxiety or depression are more prone to develop insomnia symptoms, demonstrating the intricate connection between sleep and mental health.

In conclusion, knowing the description, underlying causes, common symptoms, prevalence, and impacted demographics of insomnia is vital for recognizing and resolving this prevalent sleep problem. In the next sections of this book, we will cover options for controlling insomnia in young people, including lifestyle adjustments, cognitive-behavioral therapy, pharmaceutical therapies, and numerous home remedies targeted at encouraging restful sleep and enhancing overall well-being.

Understanding Insomnia

Insomnia is a complicated sleep condition that can be impacted by a range of circumstances. In this section, we will study the origins and contributing factors of insomnia, evaluate its gender and age distribution patterns, and give significant data regarding this widespread sleep disease.

Causes and Contributing Factors

1. Psychological Factors: Psychological problems such as stress, anxiety, sadness, and trauma can greatly contribute to sleeplessness. Persistent anxiety, racing thoughts, and emotional turmoil can

interrupt sleep patterns and contribute to trouble falling asleep or staying asleep.

2. Medical illnesses: Certain medical illnesses and health difficulties might raise the risk of sleeplessness. Chronic pain illnesses like arthritis, fibromyalgia, or migraines can create discomfort that interferes with sleep. Respiratory problems such as asthma or sleep apnea may affect breathing during sleep, resulting in frequent awakenings.

3. Lifestyle Factors: Poor sleep hygiene habits and lifestyle choices might increase insomnia symptoms. Irregular sleep patterns, excessive coffee or alcohol use, smoking, and exposure to electronic devices before bedtime can disturb the body's

normal sleep-wake cycle and affect sleep quality.

4. medicines and Substances: Some medicines, including stimulants, antidepressants, corticosteroids, and some over-the-counter pharmaceuticals, might interfere with sleep and contribute to insomnia. Additionally, drug use or withdrawal from substances like nicotine, caffeine, or alcohol can disturb sleep patterns.

5. Environmental issues: Environmental issues such as noise, light, temperature, and unpleasant bedding can interrupt sleep and lead to insomnia. Creating a sleep-friendly atmosphere with minimum distractions and

maximum comfort can encourage higher sleep quality.

6. Circadian Rhythm Disruptions: Disruptions to the body's internal clock, known as the circadian rhythm, might lead to insomnia. Shift employment, jet lag, or inconsistent sleep-wake patterns can desynchronize the body's internal clock, leading to trouble falling asleep or maintaining sleep consistency.

7. hereditary Predisposition: There may be a hereditary predisposition to insomnia, with certain individuals inheriting vulnerability to sleep problems. While genetics alone may not cause insomnia, they can combine with environmental and lifestyle variables to alter sleep patterns.

8. Stressful Life Events: Major life transitions, painful experiences, or severe stressors can provoke acute episodes of sleeplessness. Events such as job loss, marital issues, financial challenges, or bereavement can interrupt sleep patterns and increase current insomnia symptoms.

Understanding the diverse nature of insomnia and identifying potential contributing variables is vital for designing tailored treatment methods and treating underlying concerns that may be causing sleep difficulties.

Gender and Age Distribution

Insomnia can affect persons of all ages and genders, although there are noticeable trends in its occurrence across different demographic groups.

1. Gender: Research shows that women are more prone to develop insomnia compared to males. Hormonal variations throughout the menstrual cycle, pregnancy, and menopause might lead to sleep disruptions in women. Additionally, women may be more sensitive to stress-related sleep disorders due to societal duties, caregiving obligations, and hormonal changes.

2. Age: Insomnia prevalence seems to fluctuate across various age groups. While insomnia can occur at any age, it becomes more frequent with advancing age. Young people, particularly those in their late teens to early twenties, may develop transitory

insomnia owing to lifestyle issues, scholastic stress, or social demands. Middle-aged persons may encounter sleeplessness connected to work stress, family duties, or age-related health conditions. Older persons, especially those over the age of 65, may develop persistent insomnia owing to age-related changes in sleep architecture, medical comorbidities, and drug usage.

Understanding these gender and age distribution trends might guide targeted treatments and support measures geared to the individual requirements of different demographic groups impacted by insomnia.

Facts About Insomnia

1. Prevalence: Insomnia is one of the most frequent sleep disorders globally, affecting around 30% of individuals at some time in their lives. Chronic insomnia, defined as insomnia symptoms occurring at least three nights per week for three months or more affects around 10% of individuals.

2. Impact on Health: Insomnia is not only an annoyance but can have serious repercussions for physical, mental, and emotional health. Chronic insomnia is connected with an increased risk of hypertension, cardiovascular disease, diabetes, obesity, depression, anxiety disorders, and impaired immunological function. It can also affect cognitive

function, memory, focus, and decision-making ability.

3. cost Burden: Insomnia puts a major cost burden on people, healthcare institutions, and society as a whole. The direct and indirect expenses associated with insomnia-related healthcare consumption, lower job productivity, absenteeism, accidents, and concomitant health disorders lead to large financial expenditures.

4. therapy Options: Fortunately, there are effective therapy options available for controlling insomnia. These include lifestyle adjustments, cognitive-behavioral treatment for insomnia (CBT-I), pharmaceutical approaches, and complementary therapies such as relaxation methods, meditation, and

acupuncture. A multidisciplinary strategy integrating behavioral, psychological, and pharmaceutical therapies is generally suggested for optimum outcomes.

5. Quality of Life: Insomnia may dramatically impair an individual's quality of life, impacting relationships, work performance, social functioning, and general well-being. Addressing insomnia symptoms and improving sleep quality can lead to considerable gains in quality of life and functional results.

Understanding the causes, gender and age distribution trends, and critical information regarding insomnia is vital for tackling this widespread sleep condition successfully. By acknowledging the complex nature of insomnia and applying focused therapies, individuals may take proactive measures toward improving their sleep health and general quality of life.

Impact of Insomnia

Insomnia is not merely a transient nuisance; it may have substantial and long-lasting repercussions on different elements of an individual's life. In this part, we will dig into the impact of insomnia, highlighting its lifetime implications without adequate care, the physical and mental health repercussions it might entail, and its major influence on everyday functioning.

Lifetime Implications Without Proper Care

1. Chronic Health issues: Untreated insomnia can raise the chance of developing chronic health issues such as hypertension,

cardiovascular disease, diabetes, obesity, and metabolic syndrome. Prolonged sleep disorders can affect physiological functions, including hormone balance, immunological function, and glucose metabolism, leading to the genesis and worsening of these illnesses.

2. Psychological illnesses: Insomnia is directly associated with the development and worsening of several psychological illnesses, including depression, anxiety disorders, and drug use disorders. Chronic sleep deprivation can affect neurotransmitter systems involved in mood regulation, resulting in abnormalities in mood, cognition, and emotional processing.

3. shorter Life Expectancy: Long-term sleep problems have been related to an increased risk of death and shorter life expectancy. Individuals with chronic insomnia may suffer heightened stress levels, inflammation, oxidative stress, and poor physiological repair systems, which can accelerate the aging process and lead to early mortality.

4. Impaired Cognitive Function: Persistent sleep deprivation and cognitive impairment are tightly connected. Chronic insomnia can affect cognitive function, including attention, memory, executive function, and decision-making ability. Prolonged sleep disorders might hamper information processing, problem-solving skills, and general cognitive performance, hurting

academic, vocational, and social functioning.

5. Quality of Life: Insomnia may dramatically reduce an individual's quality of life, compromising physical health, mental well-being, social connections, and overall life satisfaction. Chronic sleep problems can affect daytime performance, lower energy levels, depress mood, and limit involvement in social and recreational activities, leading to poor overall quality of life.

Physical and Mental Health Consequences

1. Cardiovascular Health: Chronic insomnia is related to an increased risk of

hypertension, coronary artery disease, stroke, and heart failure. Sleep disruptions can affect cardiovascular homeostasis, leading to raised blood pressure, increased sympathetic activity, endothelial dysfunction, and inflammation, all of which contribute to cardiovascular morbidity and death.

2. Metabolic Health: Insomnia has been associated with abnormalities in glucose metabolism, insulin resistance, and dyslipidemia, raising the risk of type 2 diabetes and metabolic syndrome. Sleep deprivation can affect the balance of appetite-regulating hormones, leading to increased hunger, cravings for high-caloric meals, and weight gain, further worsening metabolic dysfunction.

3. immunological Function: Sleep plays a critical role in immunological function, with insufficient sleep impairing the body's capacity to develop an efficient immune response. Chronic insomnia is connected with abnormalities in immune cell function, greater susceptibility to infections, delayed wound healing, lengthening recovery periods, and raising the risk of infectious illnesses.

4. Mental Health: Insomnia is closely connected to several mental health issues, including depression, anxiety, bipolar disorder, and psychotic illnesses. Sleep problems can worsen existing psychiatric symptoms, provoke mood episodes, and undermine emotional control, leading to the

incidence, severity, and chronicity of mental health issues.

5. Neurological Health: Chronic sleep abnormalities have been linked to the etiology of neurodegenerative illnesses such as Alzheimer's disease and Parkinson's disease. Sleep has a vital role in brain repair, synaptic plasticity, and memory consolidation, and changes in sleep architecture can accelerate neurodegenerative processes and cognitive decline.

Impact on Daily Functioning

1. Cognitive Impairment: Insomnia can impair cognitive function, impacting attention, memory, processing speed, and

executive function. Individuals with chronic insomnia may face trouble concentrating, storing information, making judgments, and completing tasks that need prolonged concentration and mental flexibility.

2. job Performance: Sleep disorders can dramatically influence job performance, productivity, and occupational functioning. Insomnia-related tiredness, cognitive impairment, and mood disorders can affect job performance, impair decision-making abilities, raise the risk of errors and accidents, and contribute to absenteeism and presenteeism in the workplace.

3. Academic Achievement: Insomnia can interfere with academic performance and educational accomplishment, particularly

among young people and students. Sleep difficulties can affect attention, memory consolidation, and information processing, making it challenging to focus, study efficiently, and do well on examinations and assignments.

4. Social connections: Chronic sleep disorders can affect social connections and interpersonal interactions. Insomnia-related irritation, mood swings, and weariness can impact communication, emotional expression, and conflict resolution, leading to interpersonal disputes, social retreat, and feelings of isolation and loneliness.

5. Quality of Life: Insomnia can reduce overall quality of life, affecting physical health, mental well-being, social

connections, and everyday functioning. Persistent sleep problems can impede enjoyment of leisure activities, limit participation in social gatherings, and lower life satisfaction, leading to emotions of frustration, powerlessness, and impaired quality of life.

Insomnia can have far-reaching effects on an individual's physical health, emotional well-being, and everyday functioning. Understanding the tremendous impact of insomnia underlines the significance of early detection, quick intervention, and comprehensive treatment measures to limit its adverse impacts and promote overall well-being.

Diagnosis and Evaluation

Insomnia, though frequent and disruptive, is a very curable disorder when detected and handled effectively. This section digs into the diagnostic procedure for insomnia, revealing the essential processes required in recognizing symptoms and completing a medical examination to discover the underlying causes and contributing variables.

Identifying Symptoms

1. Subjective Complaints: The diagnostic path generally starts with the patient's subjective complaints regarding their sleep patterns and experiences. Individuals with

insomnia often report problems getting asleep, remaining asleep, or enduring non-restorative sleep despite enough chance for rest.

2. length and Frequency: Clinicians examine the length and frequency of sleep disruptions reported by the patient. Insomnia is characterized by chronic sleep problems that occur at least three nights per week and last for at least three months, adversely impairing daytime functioning and overall quality of life.

3. Daytime Symptoms: Insomnia is commonly accompanied by a multitude of daytime symptoms, including tiredness, drowsiness, irritability, emotional problems, cognitive impairment, and decreased

occupational or academic functioning. These daytime symptoms may be suggestive of underlying sleep disorders and demand further assessment.

4. Sleep Diary: Patients may be requested to maintain a sleep diary to document their sleep-wake cycles, bedtime rituals, sleep onset latency, total sleep duration, nocturnal awakenings, and daily functioning during a given period. Sleep diaries give useful insights into the nature and severity of sleep problems and assist guide diagnostic and therapy decisions.

5. Assessment methods: Clinicians may apply standardized assessment methods, such as the Pittsburgh Sleep Quality Index (PSQI) or the Insomnia Severity Index (ISI),

to quantify the severity of insomnia symptoms and measure the impact on several areas of functioning. These diagnostic methods let doctors evaluate the subjective experience of insomnia and follow treatment effects over time.

Medical Evaluation Process

1. Complete History: The medical assessment method begins with a complete history-taking to explicate the patient's sleep patterns, bedtime rituals, sleep environment, prior medical history, mental history, medication usage, drug use, and psychosocial stresses. A detailed grasp of the patient's medical and psychological background helps uncover potential

predisposing, precipitating, and perpetuating variables leading to insomnia.

2. Physical Examination: A full physical examination may be undertaken to screen for evidence of medical diseases or comorbidities contributing to sleep difficulties. Physical examination abnormalities, such as obesity, hypertension, or symptoms of obstructive sleep apnea (OSA), may merit additional assessment and management.

3. Laboratory studies: In select situations, laboratory studies may be suggested to screen for underlying medical diseases linked with sleep difficulties. These investigations may involve blood tests to measure thyroid function, metabolic

parameters, inflammatory markers, or other biochemical parameters relevant to the patient's clinical presentation.

4. Sleep Studies: Polysomnography (PSG) or home sleep apnea testing (HSAT) may be advised when there is suspicion of concomitant sleep disorders, such as obstructive sleep apnea, periodic limb movement disorder, or REM sleep behavior disorder. These sleep investigations assist examine sleep architecture, respiratory characteristics, nocturnal movements, and other physiological factors to clarify the underlying processes contributing to sleep problems.

5. Psychological Evaluation: To assess mood symptoms, anxiety symptoms, cognitive

distortions, maladaptive coping mechanisms, and psychosocial stressors causing insomnia, a psychological evaluation may be necessary for individuals with coexisting psychiatric disorders or psychological distress. Psychological examinations assist in customized therapies to address underlying psychological causes causing sleep difficulties.

6. Collaborative Approach: The diagnostic examination of insomnia typically involves a collaborative approach involving primary care doctors, sleep experts, psychiatrists, psychologists, and other healthcare professionals. Collaborative decision-making guarantees full assessment, accurate diagnosis, and individualized

treatment regimens addressing the multidimensional character of insomnia.

The diagnosis approach for insomnia comprises a detailed review of the patient's sleep problems, daytime functioning, medical history, physical examination results, and, where warranted, laboratory tests, sleep studies, and psychological assessments. A full knowledge of the underlying variables leading to insomnia is crucial for directing tailored treatment options and enhancing clinical results.

Management and Treatment

Insomnia, a frequent sleep condition characterized by difficulty getting asleep, staying asleep, or having non-restorative sleep, can greatly impact an individual's quality of life and general well-being. Effective management and treatment options have a vital role in reducing insomnia symptoms, increasing sleep quality, and promoting daytime performance. This section discusses several techniques for controlling and treating insomnia, spanning lifestyle adjustments, cognitive-behavioral therapy (CBT), and pharmaceutical therapies.

Lifestyle Modifications

1. Sleep Hygiene Practices: Implementing appropriate sleep hygiene practices is crucial in supporting good sleep habits and enhancing sleep quality. Recommendations include maintaining a consistent sleep

schedule, providing a suitable sleep environment that is dark, quiet, and comfortable, avoiding stimulating activities before bedtime, reducing coffee and alcohol intake, and participating in relaxation techniques to decompress before sleep.

2. Stress Management: Effective stress management practices, such as mindfulness meditation, progressive muscle relaxation, deep breathing exercises, and yoga, can help decrease anxiety and improve relaxation, hence aiding sleep onset and maintenance. Incorporating stress-reduction methods into daily routines helps lessen the influence of stress on sleep quality and general well-being.

3. Regular Exercise: Engaging in regular physical exercise, ideally earlier in the day, offers several health advantages, including increased sleep quality and sleep efficiency. Aerobic activity, weight training, or flexibility exercises undertaken regularly can increase sleep architecture, reduce sleep latency, and boost total sleep continuity. However, excessive exercise close to bedtime should be avoided since it may interfere with sleep beginning.

4. Healthy Diet and Nutrition: Adopting a balanced diet rich in fruits, vegetables, whole grains, lean meats, and healthy fats enhances general health and may significantly affect sleep quality. Avoiding heavy or spicy meals, caffeine, and large quantities of fluids close to bedtime might

minimize stomach discomfort and nocturnal awakenings, supporting unbroken sleep.

5. Limiting Screen Time: Electronic gadgets, such as smartphones, tablets, and laptops, produce blue light that can suppress melatonin synthesis and disturb circadian cycles, thus reducing sleep quality. Limiting screen time before bedtime and adopting blue light filters or "night mode" settings on electronic devices might lessen the detrimental effects of blue light exposure on sleep.

6. Establishing a soothing Bedtime Routine: Establishing a soothing bedtime routine indicates to the body that it is time to wind down and prepare for sleep. Engaging in relaxing activities, such as reading, listening

to soothing music, having a warm bath, or practicing relaxation methods, can induce relaxation and assist the transition to sleep.

Cognitive-behavioral therapy (CBT)

1. Overview: Cognitive-behavioral therapy for insomnia (CBT-I) is a systematic, evidence-based treatment method targeted at resolving maladaptive thoughts, actions, and beliefs linked with insomnia. CBT-I tackles the cognitive and behavioral variables leading to sleep disruptions, allowing individuals to establish healthy sleep habits and attitudes towards sleep.

2. Components of CBT-I: CBT-I generally involves multiple components, including cognitive restructuring, stimulus control

treatment, sleep restriction therapy, relaxation methods, and sleep hygiene instruction. These components are designed to match the distinct requirements and preferences of each individual, enabling lasting gains in sleep quality and daytime performance.

3. Cognitive Restructuring: Cognitive restructuring includes recognizing and addressing negative or unreasonable attitudes and beliefs about sleep that lead to insomnia. Through cognitive restructuring strategies, individuals learn to replace maladaptive sleep-related cognitions with more realistic and adaptive alternatives, lowering anxiety and stress around sleep.

4. Stimulus Control treatment: Stimulus control treatment tries to reassociate the bed and bedroom surroundings with sleep and relaxation rather than awake and arousal. This entails setting rigorous sleep-wake patterns, utilizing the bed solely for sleep and sexual activity, and participating in calming activities outside the bedroom if unable to fall asleep within a certain time limit.

5. Sleep Restriction treatment: Sleep restriction treatment seeks to consolidate sleep by restricting time spent in bed to match the individual's real sleep length. By progressively lowering time spent in bed and gradually boosting sleep efficiency, sleep restriction treatment helps enhance

sleep continuity and promote more restorative sleep.

6. Relaxation methods: Incorporating relaxation methods, such as progressive muscle relaxation, deep breathing exercises, guided imagery, and mindfulness meditation, into nighttime rituals can lower physiological arousal, relieve anxiety, and promote relaxation favorable to sleep onset.

7. Sleep Hygiene Education: Sleep hygiene education entails teaching individuals about good sleep habits and activities favorable to optimal sleep quality. Topics may include maintaining a consistent sleep schedule, providing a pleasant sleep environment, avoiding stimulants before bedtime, and

practicing relaxation techniques to improve sleep.

8. Effectiveness of CBT-I: Research suggests that CBT-I is extremely successful in treating insomnia and is related to persistent improvements in sleep quality, reduced sleep latency, fewer nocturnal awakenings, and increased daytime functioning. CBT-I is indicated as the first-line treatment for chronic insomnia and is typically favored over pharmaceutical therapies due to its long-term effectiveness and benign side-effect profile.

Pharmacological Interventions

1. Overview: Pharmacological therapies are widely employed in the therapy of insomnia and widely employed in the therapy of insomnia

to offer symptomatic relief and enhance sleep initiation and maintenance. While medication may be effective for the short-term treatment of insomnia, long-term usage is typically contraindicated due to the possibility of tolerance, reliance, and side effects.

2. Types of pharmaceuticals: Pharmacological drugs often used in the treatment of insomnia include sedative-hypnotic pharmaceuticals, such as benzodiazepines, non-benzodiazepine hypnotics, melatonin receptor agonists, and antidepressants with sedating effects. These drugs exert their effects via regulating neurotransmitter systems involved in sleep regulation, such as gamma-aminobutyric acid (GABA) and melatonin.

3. Benzodiazepines: Benzodiazepines, such as temazepam, lorazepam, and diazepam, are central nervous system depressants that augment the inhibitory effects of GABA, resulting in drowsiness and anxiolysis. While useful for short-term treatment of insomnia, benzodiazepines entail a risk of tolerance, dependency, withdrawal, and side effects, such as daytime sedation, cognitive impairment, and motor dysfunction.

4. Non-Benzodiazepine Hypnotics: Non-benzodiazepine hypnotics, including zolpidem, zaleplon, and eszopiclone, preferentially target the benzodiazepine receptor subtype within the GABA-A receptor complex, exerting sedative and hypnotic effects. Non-benzodiazepine hypnotics are linked with a decreased risk of

dependency and withdrawal compared to benzodiazepines but may still induce unpleasant effects, such as next-day sleepiness, dizziness, and cognitive impairment.

5. Melatonin Receptor Agonists: Melatonin receptor agonists, such as ramelteon and tasimelteon, target melatonin receptors in the suprachiasmatic nucleus of the hypothalamus, regulating circadian rhythms and encouraging sleep onset. Melatonin receptor agonists are typically well-tolerated and have no risk of dependency or withdrawal but may induce transitory dizziness, headache, and weariness.

6. Antidepressants: Certain antidepressants, such as trazodone, amitriptyline, and Pepin

contain sedating effects and are occasionally used off-label in the treatment of insomnia, particularly in persons with concomitant depression or anxiety. These antidepressants produce their calming effects by diverse mechanisms, including blockage of histamine receptors, serotonin reuptake inhibition, and antagonism of alpha-adrenergic receptors.

7. Personalized Therapy Approach: The degree of sleeplessness, coexisting medical or mental health issues, medication tolerability, possible drug interactions, and patient preferences should all be taken into consideration when choosing pharmacological treatments for insomnia. Clinicians must consider the advantages and dangers of pharmacotherapy and engage in

collaborative decision-making with patients to improve treatment results while reducing unwanted effects.

The management and treatment of insomnia entail a complex strategy comprising lifestyle adjustments, cognitive-behavioral therapy, and pharmaceutical therapies customized to fit the particular requirements and preferences of each individual. By employing evidence-based techniques and building a collaborative therapeutic alliance between patients and healthcare providers, insomnia can be effectively controlled, leading to increased sleep quality, greater daytime functioning, and overall well-being.

8 Home Remedies for Insomnia

Insomnia, a frequent sleep condition characterized by difficulty getting asleep, staying asleep, or having non-restorative sleep, can dramatically influence an individual's quality of life and general well-being. While pharmaceutical medications and behavioral therapies are routinely applied to address insomnia, many individuals prefer natural and holistic ways to enhance sleep quality. This section discusses eight home treatments for insomnia, spanning mindfulness meditation, mantra repetition, yoga, exercise, massage, magnesium supplements, lavender oil, and melatonin supplementation.

Mindfulness Meditation

Mindfulness meditation, founded in ancient contemplative traditions, has earned broad attention for its capacity to ease stress, induce relaxation, and enhance sleep quality. Mindfulness meditation entails building present-moment awareness via focused attention on breath, physical sensations, thoughts, and emotions without judgment. By fostering a non-reactive awareness of internal and external sensations, individuals can minimize rumination, anxiety, and physiological arousal, helping the transition to sleep.

Research suggests that regular mindfulness meditation practice is connected with benefits in sleep latency, sleep efficiency, and overall sleep quality. A 2015 research published in JAMA Internal Medicine demonstrated that mindfulness meditation significantly improved insomnia symptoms and sleep quality in older individuals compared to sleep hygiene instruction alone. Incorporating mindfulness meditation into evening practices can help individuals unwind, quiet the mind, and develop a sense of calm conducive to deep sleep.

Mantra Repetition

Mantra repetition, a centuries-old spiritual practice coming from Hindu and Buddhist traditions, comprises the silent or audible repetition of a holy word, phrase, or sound known as a mantra. Mantra repetition acts as a focus point for attention, helping individuals to acquire concentration, inner tranquility, and spiritual connection. By saying a mantra with intention and commitment, individuals can calm the mind, eliminate mental chatter, and produce a state of profound relaxation suitable for sleep.

Studies have established the usefulness of mantra repetition in lowering insomnia symptoms and enhancing sleep quality. A 2015 research published in the Journal of Evidence-Based Complementary & Alternative Medicine explored the effects of mantra repetition on sleep quality in women facing homelessness. The study indicated that participants who performed mantra repetition reported substantial improvements in insomnia symptoms and perceived stress levels compared to those in the control group. Incorporating mantra repetition into bedtime rituals can help individuals unwind, reduce tension, and smooth the transition to deep sleep.

Yoga

Yoga, an ancient mind-body practice originating from India, blends physical postures, breathwork, and meditation to achieve comprehensive health and well-being. Yoga activities, such as asanas (physical postures), pranayama (breath control), and dhyana (meditation), assist individuals acquire awareness, balance, and relaxation. By coordinating breath with movement and promoting awareness, yoga promotes physiological and psychological relaxation, helping the transition to sleep.

Numerous research have proved the therapeutic effects of yoga on sleep quality and insomnia symptoms. A 2014 systematic study published in the Journal of Clinical Psychology study studied the effects of yoga on sleep quality in adults. The review indicated that yoga treatments were related to improvements in sleep metrics, including sleep latency, sleep length, and sleep efficiency. Incorporating mild, restorative yoga techniques before bedtime can help individuals release tension, calm the mind, and prepare the body for restorative sleep.

Exercise

Regular exercise is a cornerstone of a healthy lifestyle and is connected with several physical and mental health benefits, including increased sleep quality and insomnia management. Engaging in aerobic activity, weight training, or flexibility exercises regularly helps regulate circadian cycles, lower stress hormones, and increase relaxation, all of which lead to better sleep quality.

Studies have repeatedly established the positive benefits of exercise on sleep quality and insomnia symptoms. A 2015 research published in the journal Sleep Medicine Reviews studied the influence of exercise on sleep in middle-aged and older persons. The study indicated that regular exercise was related to improvements in many sleep metrics, including sleep length, sleep efficiency, and sleep start latency. Incorporating moderate-intensity exercise into daily routines, particularly earlier in the day, can assist individuals manage sleep-wake cycles, minimize sleep disruptions, and boost overall sleep quality.

Massage

Massage therapy, characterized by the manipulation of soft tissues and muscles, is generally acknowledged for its capacity to induce relaxation, ease muscle tension, and lower stress levels. Massage treatment activates the parasympathetic nervous system, prompting the production of endorphins and fostering a state of profound relaxation conducive to sleep. By targeting areas of tension and increasing circulation, massage therapy can ease physical discomfort and create emotions of relaxation and well-being, aiding the transition to sleep.

Numerous studies have established the therapeutic effects of massage treatment on sleep quality and insomnia symptoms. A 2015 meta-analysis published in the journal Sleep Medicine Reviews investigated the efficacy of massage treatment for improving sleep quality in adults. The meta-analysis indicated that massage treatment was related to significant increases in subjective sleep quality and decreases in insomnia symptoms. Incorporating self-massage techniques or seeking professional massage therapy sessions can help individuals relax, unwind, and prepare for restful sleep.

Magnesium Supplementation

Magnesium, an important element involved in over 300 metabolic activities in the body, plays a critical role in regulating neurotransmitter activity, muscular relaxation, and stress response. Magnesium shortage has been associated with insomnia, anxiety, and restless leg syndrome, underscoring the necessity of appropriate magnesium intake for fostering healthy sleep patterns. Supplementation with magnesium may assist individuals relax, relieve muscular tension, and aid sleep onset and maintenance.

Research shows that magnesium supplementation may be effective in increasing sleep quality and lowering insomnia symptoms. A 2012 research published in the Journal of Research in Medical Sciences explored the effects of magnesium supplementation on insomnia symptoms in older persons. The study indicated that people who got magnesium supplementation had increases in sleep efficiency, sleep duration, and sleep start latency compared to those in the control group. Incorporating magnesium-rich foods, such as leafy greens, nuts, seeds, and whole grains, or taking magnesium supplements under the advice of a healthcare expert can promote good sleep patterns and general well-being.

Lavender Oil

Lavender oil, produced from the lavender plant, is recognized for its relaxing and sedative effects, making it a popular cure for encouraging relaxation and enhancing sleep quality. Lavender oil includes linalool and linalyl acetate, chemicals that exert anxiolytic, sedative, and mood-stabilizing actions on the central nervous system. Inhalation or topical use of lavender oil can trigger sensations of relaxation, lower anxiety levels, and increase sleep start and duration.

Numerous studies have proved the therapeutic effects of lavender oil on sleep quality and insomnia symptoms. A 2014 research published in the journal

Evidence-Based Complementary and Alternative Medicine explored the impact of lavender oil aromatherapy on sleep quality in individuals with depression. The study indicated that those who received lavender oil inhalation had substantial improvements in sleep quality and insomnia severity compared to those in the control group. Incorporating lavender oil into nighttime routines, such as diffusing lavender oil in the bedroom or adding a few drops to a warm bath, can improve relaxation, induce sleep, and boost overall sleep quality.

Melatonin Supplementation

Melatonin, a hormone released by the pineal gland in reaction to darkness, plays a critical function in regulating the sleep-wake cycle and encouraging sleep onset. Melatonin levels normally rise in the evening, signaling to the body that it is time to sleep, and fall in the morning upon exposure to light. Supplementing with melatonin can assist regulate circadian rhythms, induce drowsiness, and enhance sleep quality, particularly in persons with circadian rhythm problems or jet lag.

Research shows that melatonin supplementation may be effective in enhancing sleep quality and lowering insomnia symptoms. A 2016 research published in the journal Supportive Care in Cancer explored the impact of melatonin supplementation on sleep patterns in cancer patients with insomnia. The study indicated that those who got melatonin supplementation saw substantial increases in sleep quality, sleep latency, and sleep duration compared to those in the control group. Incorporating melatonin supplementation under the advice of a healthcare practitioner can help patients manage sleep-wake cycles, minimize insomnia symptoms, and boost overall sleep quality.

In conclusion, including these eight home remedies for insomnia in daily routines will help individuals increase relaxation, decrease tension, and enhance sleep quality organically. By adopting comprehensive methods of sleep management, individuals may establish good sleep habits, boost sleep quality, and promote overall well-being. However, it is vital to speak with a healthcare practitioner before commencing any new sleep treatments, especially if you have underlying health concerns or are taking drugs that may interfere with these cures.

Tips for Better Sleep

Quality sleep is vital for general health and well-being. However, many individuals deal with insomnia or poor sleep quality owing to several causes, including stress, lifestyle behaviors, and environmental influences. Incorporating simple yet effective measures for improved sleep can greatly enhance sleep quality and overall health. In this part, we will discuss practical suggestions and practices to boost sleep quality and promote restorative sleep.

Healthy Sleep Habits

1. Establish a Bedtime Routine: Consistency is crucial to supporting healthy sleep habits.

Establish a soothing nighttime ritual to communicate to your body that it is time to wind down and prepare for sleep. This may include things such as reading a book, having a warm bath, or practicing relaxation techniques like deep breathing or meditation.

2. Create a Sleep-Friendly Environment: Your sleep environment plays a significant part in influencing sleep quality. Make sure your bedroom is cold, dark, and quiet to encourage good sleep. Invest in comfortable bedding and pillows that assist in appropriate spinal alignment and increase comfort.

3. Limit Screen Time Before Bed: Exposure to blue light generated by electronic devices

such as smartphones, tablets, and laptops can interfere with the synthesis of melatonin, a hormone that governs sleep-wake cycles. Avoid screen time at least an hour before bedtime to encourage relaxation and increase sleep quality.

4. Avoid Stimulants Before Bed: Caffeine, nicotine, and alcohol can alter sleep patterns and lead to insomnia. Limit the use of caffeinated beverages such as coffee, tea, and soda in the afternoon and evening, and avoid alcohol and nicotine close to bedtime.

5. Manage Stress: Chronic stress and worry can interfere with sleep quality and lead to insomnia. Practice stress-reduction strategies such as mindfulness meditation, deep breathing exercises, or progressive

muscle relaxation to improve relaxation and decrease tension before bedtime.

Creating a Conducive Sleep Environment

1. Optimize Bedroom Conditions: Your bedroom environment plays a significant part in encouraging good sleep. Keep your bedroom cold, dark, and quiet to produce an optimal sleep environment. Use blackout curtains or eye masks to block off light, and try using white noise generators or earplugs to conceal disturbing sounds.

2. Invest in a Comfortable Mattress and Bedding: Your mattress and bedding may greatly affect sleep quality and comfort. Choose a mattress and pillows that give

appropriate support for your body and encourage good spinal alignment. Invest in high-quality bedding constructed from breathable, natural materials to boost comfort and encourage peaceful sleep.

3. Minimize Clutter: A messy bedroom may add to emotions of tension and worry, making it difficult to relax and unwind before bedtime. Keep your bedroom tidy, orderly, and free of clutter to produce a tranquil sleep environment conducive to peaceful sleep.

4. Control Temperature: Temperature may have a substantial influence on sleep quality. Keep your bedroom cold and comfy, ideally between 60 to 67 degrees Fahrenheit (15 to 19 degrees Celsius), to encourage peaceful

sleep. Use fans or air conditioning to maintain a comfortable temperature, and consider using breathable mattress fabrics to minimize overheating.

Establishing a Consistent Sleep Schedule

1. Maintain a Regular Sleep-Wake Schedule: Consistency is crucial to supporting good sleep habits. Go to bed and wake up at the same time every day, including on weekends, to regulate your body's internal clock and encourage peaceful sleep. Avoid napping late in the day, since this might interfere with your ability to fall asleep at night.

2. Limit Daytime Naps: While brief daytime naps might be useful for some individuals, excessive or extended napping can disturb evening sleep patterns and lead to insomnia. Limit daytime naps to 20-30 minutes and avoid sleeping late in the day to encourage improved sleep quality at night.

3. Expose Yourself to Natural Light: Exposure to natural light during the day helps regulate your body's internal clock and supports healthy sleep-wake cycles. Spend time outside during the day, particularly in the morning, to expose oneself to natural light to increase alertness and mood during the day, and encourage peaceful sleep at night.

Managing Stress and Anxiety

1. Practice Relaxation methods: Relaxation methods such as deep breathing, progressive muscle relaxation, and guided imagery can help decrease tension and promote relaxation before bedtime. Incorporate relaxation activities into your nighttime routine to calm the mind and prepare for sleep.

2. Limit Stimulating Activities Before Bed: Engaging in stimulating activities such as work-related duties, strenuous exercise, or emotionally charged talks before bedtime can boost arousal levels and make it difficult to fall asleep. Avoid stimulating activities at least an hour before bedtime to encourage relaxation and prepare for sleep.

3. Create a Worry notebook: If racing thoughts or anxieties keep you up at night, consider maintaining a worry notebook to jot down your thoughts and concerns before bedtime. Writing down your problems can help you organize your thoughts and emotions and decrease anxiety, making it easier to relax and go to sleep.

4. Seek assistance: If stress or worry is interfering with your ability to sleep, don't hesitate to seek assistance from a mental health professional. Therapy, counseling, or cognitive-behavioral therapy (CBT) can help you build coping techniques, handle stress more effectively, and improve sleep quality.

Caregiving and Support

Supporting persons with insomnia entails recognizing their particular requirements, giving emotional support, promoting adherence to treatment regimens, and offering aid with lifestyle improvements. Caregivers play a significant role in helping people manage insomnia and improve their sleep quality. In this part, we will cover ways of for caring and supporting persons with insomnia.

Understanding the Needs of Individuals with Insomnia

1. Listen and affirm: The first step in offering effective assistance is to listen to the

individual's problems and affirm their experiences. Insomnia may be a tough and stressful illness, and individuals may feel irritated, nervous, or despairing about their sleep troubles. By listening attentively and respecting their feelings, caregivers may create a supportive atmosphere where people feel understood and appreciated.

2. Educate Yourself: Take the time to educate yourself on insomnia, its origins, symptoms, and treatment choices. Understanding the nature of the disease can help caregivers offer educated assistance and aid clients in navigating their road toward healthier sleep.

3. Be Empathetic: Show empathy and compassion towards persons battling with

sleeplessness. Recognize that sleep disorders can have a substantial influence on their physical and emotional well-being, as well as their quality of life. Offer comfort and sympathy, and avoid underestimating or disregarding their experiences.

4. Encourage Open Communication: Encourage individuals to freely share their issues, preferences, and requirements surrounding their sleep. Create a secure and non-judgmental atmosphere where people feel comfortable addressing their issues with insomnia, as well as any challenges they may find during therapy.

Providing Emotional Support

1. Offer Emotional Validation: Validate the individual's feelings and experiences connected to sleeplessness. Let them know that their sentiments are real and reasonable, and comfort them that they are not alone in their challenges.

2. Be a Good Listener: Practice active listening and give a supporting presence for folks to discuss their ideas and feelings regarding their sleep troubles. Avoid delivering unsolicited advice or trying to "fix" their problems; instead, focus on empathic listening and acknowledging their experiences.

3. Provide Encouragement: Offer words of encouragement and support to folks as they navigate their road towards improved sleep. Celebrate their accomplishments, no matter how modest, and remind them that beneficial changes require time and work.

4. Give practical aid: In addition to emotional support, give practical aid to persons battling with sleeplessness. This may involve helping them with everyday duties, giving transportation to medical appointments, or aiding with domestic chores to ease stress and encourage relaxation.

Encouraging Adherence to Treatment Plans

1. Discuss Treatment choices: Work cooperatively with patients to explore multiple treatment choices for insomnia, including lifestyle adjustments, therapy, and medication. Discuss the possible advantages and hazards of each treatment, and help them make educated decisions regarding their care.

2. Address hurdles to Adherence: Identify any hurdles or challenges that may prevent patients from sticking to their treatment regimens, such as financial restrictions, lack of social support, or worries about side effects. Work collaboratively to identify

solutions and overcome these challenges to maintain continuity of care.

3. Provide Gentle Reminders: Offer gentle reminders and encouragement to folks to follow through with their treatment programs. Help them build routines and ways to incorporate their therapy into their daily life efficiently.

4. Monitor Progress: Regularly monitor and analyze people's progress with their treatment programs. Check-in with them frequently to see how they are feeling and whether they are experiencing any improvements or setbacks. Adjust treatment tactics as appropriate based on their input and reaction to treatments.

Offering Assistance with Lifestyle Modifications

1. Promote Healthy Sleep Practices: Educate persons about the need to adopt healthy sleep practices to enhance sleep quality. Offer advice on developing a consistent sleep routine, generating a suitable sleep environment, and practicing relaxation methods before bedtime.

2. Encourage Physical exercise: Encourage individuals to engage in regular physical exercise, as it can assist promote improved sleep quality and general well-being. Suggest adding exercise into their regular routinc, but warn against excessive activity close to bedtime, since it may interfere with sleep.

3. Provide Nutritional advice: Offer nutritional advice and help clients in adopting good eating choices that promote better sleep. Encourage them to avoid coffee, nicotine, and heavy meals close to bedtime, and highlight the significance of ingesting sleep-promoting foods such as fruits, vegetables, and whole grains.

4. Support Stress Management: Help individuals establish effective stress management skills to minimize anxiety and enhance calm. Encourage activities such as mindfulness meditation, deep breathing exercises, and progressive muscle relaxation to help individuals cope with stress and enhance sleep quality.

Caregivers play a critical role in assisting patients with insomnia by recognizing their requirements, giving emotional support, promoting adherence to treatment programs, and offering aid with lifestyle adaptations. By delivering compassionate care and practical support, caregivers may help persons manage their sleep challenges and enhance their overall quality of life.

Conclusion

Throughout this thorough guide, we have addressed numerous elements of insomnia, including its description, causes, symptoms, diagnosis, management, and caregiving practices. Here is a review of the important themes discussed:

Insomnia is a common sleep problem characterized by trouble getting asleep, staying asleep, or both, which can profoundly influence an individual's physical and emotional well-being.

The reasons for insomnia are diverse and may include psychological problems, medical disorders, lifestyle behaviors, and environmental variables.

Common symptoms of insomnia include trouble falling asleep, waking up repeatedly during the night, waking up too early in the morning, and feeling unrefreshed upon awakening.

Diagnosis of insomnia often entails a comprehensive review of symptoms, medical history, and sleep habits, frequently including a physical exam and even sleep tests.

Management of insomnia comprises lifestyle adjustments, cognitive-behavioral therapy (CBT), pharmaceutical therapies, and home cures.

Caregivers play a critical role in assisting patients with insomnia by recognizing their requirements, giving emotional support, promoting adherence to treatment programs, and offering aid with lifestyle adaptations.

Importance of Seeking Professional Help

While self-care measures and home remedies can be effective for treating minor insomnia, it is crucial to underline the significance of obtaining professional treatment for chronic or severe sleep disorders. Professional healthcare practitioners, including physicians, sleep specialists, psychologists, and therapists, can give specialized examinations, diagnoses, and treatment choices tailored to the individual's particular needs.

Ignoring chronic insomnia or depending entirely on over-the-counter medicines without expert assistance may lead to worsened symptoms, lower quality of life, and serious problems. Therefore, those facing persistent sleep disorders should not hesitate to seek help from trained healthcare specialists to handle their concerns efficiently.

Empowering Individuals to Manage Insomnia Effectively

Empowerment sits at the foundation of good insomnia management. By teaching individuals about the nature of insomnia, its probable causes, and accessible treatment choices, we empower them to take an active part in their sleep health. Encouraging self-awareness, self-care practices, and self-advocacy helps individuals make educated decisions about their sleep and seek appropriate support when required.

Furthermore, encouraging individuals to prioritize their sleep and prioritize self-care develops a sense of agency and control over their well-being. By developing good sleep habits, exercising stress management strategies, and getting professional treatment when required, individuals may recover control over their sleep and enhance their entire quality of life.

Resources for Further Assistance and Support

In addition to professional healthcare experts, individuals seeking extra aid and support for insomnia can benefit from many resources and organizations dedicated to sleep health. These resources may include:

1. National Sleep Foundation: A non-profit organization committed to promoting sleep health and well-being through education, advocacy, and research. The National Sleep Foundation offers extensive information, suggestions, and resources on sleep problems, including insomnia.

2. American Academy of Sleep Medicine (AASM): A professional association focused

on sleep medicine and sleep research. The AASM provides helpful resources for those seeking information about sleep disorders, including insomnia, as well as directories for identifying licensed sleep facilities and board-certified sleep experts.

3. Online Support Groups and Forums: Online communities and support groups can give individuals a platform to interact with others suffering similar sleep issues, exchange experiences, and offer mutual support and encouragement. Websites such as Inspire, Sleep Disorders Guide, and Reddit's r/insomnia are examples of online communities where users may find support and solidarity.

4. Books and Publications: Numerous books, articles, and publications are available that give in-depth information and practical recommendations for controlling insomnia. Some recommended titles are "The Insomnia Workbook" by Stephanie Silberman, "No More Sleepless Nights" by Peter Hauri and Shirley Linde, and "The Sleep Solution" by Chris Winter, MD.

By accessing these tools and getting support from experienced specialists, individuals may receive the guidance, information, and assistance they need to effectively manage their insomnia and enhance their sleep quality and overall well-being. Remember, you are not alone in your quest towards improved sleep, and aid is there to support you every step of the way.

In conclusion, insomnia is a widespread and frequently problematic sleep disorder that can greatly influence an individual's quality of life. However, with correct awareness, support, and therapy, individuals may learn to manage their insomnia efficiently and recover control over their sleep health. By prioritizing self-care, getting professional help when required, and using accessible resources and support networks, individuals may begin on a road toward better sleep and greater well-being.